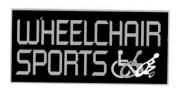

Wheelchair Basketball

by Stan Labanowich

Content Consultant:

Robert J. Szyman, Ph.D.
Youth Division Commissioner
National Wheelchair Basketball Association

RiverFront Books

An Imprint of Franklin Watts
A Division of Grolier Publishing
New York   London   Hong Kong   Sydney
Danbury, Connecticut

RiverFront Books
http://publishing.grolier.com
Copyright © 1998 by Capstone Press. All rights reserved.
Published simultaneously in Canada.
Printed in the United States of America.

Library of Congress Cataloging-in-Publication Data

Labanowich, Stan.
    Wheelchair basketball / by Stan Labanowich
    p. c.m. — (Wheelchair sports)
    Includes bibliographical references (p. 42) and index.
    Summary: Discusses the history, rules, equipment, and training
related to wheelchair basketball.
    ISBN 1-56065-614-X
    1. Wheelchair basketball—Juvenile literature. [1. Wheelchair
basketball. 2. Sports for the physically handicapped.] I. Title.
II. Series.
GV886.5.L33 1997
796.323'8—dc21
                                                              97-19254
                                                                  CIP
                                                                   AC

Editorial Credits
Editor, Greg Linder; cover design and logo, Timothy Halldin; photo
research, Michelle L. Norstad
Photo Credits
Canadian Wheelchair Basketball Association, 32-33
Index Stock/Ellen Skye, 28
Sports 'N Spokes/Paralyzed Veterans of America, 4, 36; Curt
    Beamer, 12, 17, 20, 26, 30, 34, 38; Curt Beamer and Delfina
    Colby, 8-9; Delfina Colby, cover, 23, 24
Unicorn Stock/Jean Higgins, 6, 14, 18; Aneal S. Vohra, 10;
    Betts Anderson, 43; Dennis MacDonald, 47

Special thanks to *Sports 'N Spokes*/Parlyzed Veterans of America
    and Wheelchair Sports, USA.

Table of Contents

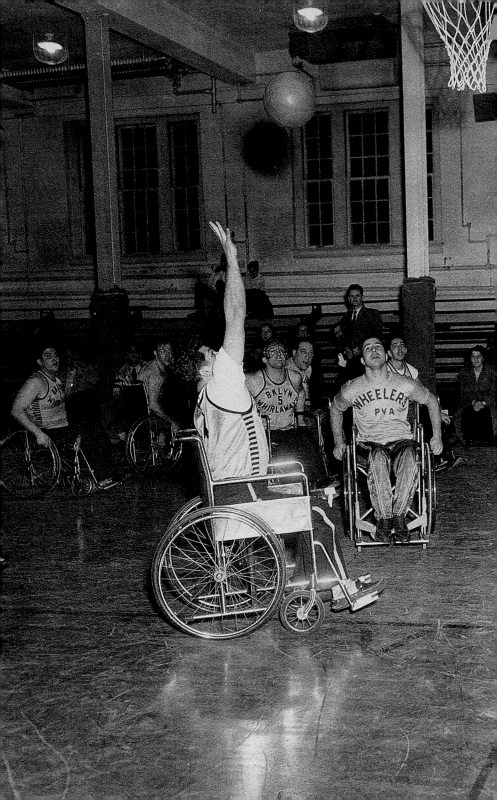

Chapter 1
Wheelchair Basketball

In 1891, Dr. James Naismith invented a new sport. The game was designed for his students at the YMCA Training School in Springfield, Massachusetts. The new sport was called basketball. Wheelchair basketball is the same sport, but it is played by people in wheelchairs.

The first basketball players threw a soccer ball into peach baskets. The baskets hung from a balcony. When a player made a successful shot, the ball stayed in the basket. Someone had to climb a ladder to get the ball back.

Basketball has changed since it was invented in 1891.

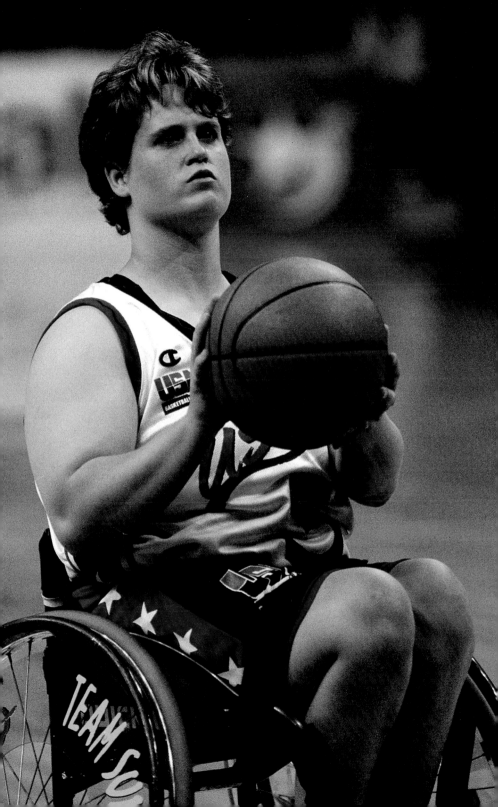

Basketball changed quickly. By 1893, metal hoops were used instead of wooden baskets. In 1895, a board was placed behind the hoop. Missed shots bounced off the backboard. Players fought to get rebounds. A rebound is when a player grabs the ball after a missed shot.

Wheelchair basketball was invented during World War II (1939-1945). Near the end of the war, wounded soldiers filled hospitals around the world. Thousands of these hospital patients could not move around without using wheelchairs.

Many of the hospitals had gyms. Patients in wheelchairs started shooting baskets. The first wheelchair basketball game was played in California in 1945. Before long, the sport turned into a new kind of basketball.

Wheelchair basketball is the most popular sport for people with disabilities. A person with disabilities is someone who has a permanent illness, injury, or birth defect. The sport is now played in more than 75 countries.

Wheelchair basketball is the most popular sport for people with disabilities.

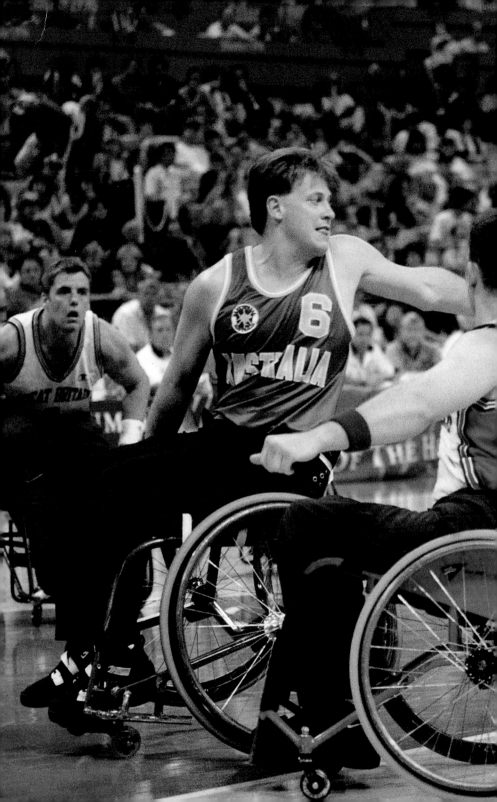

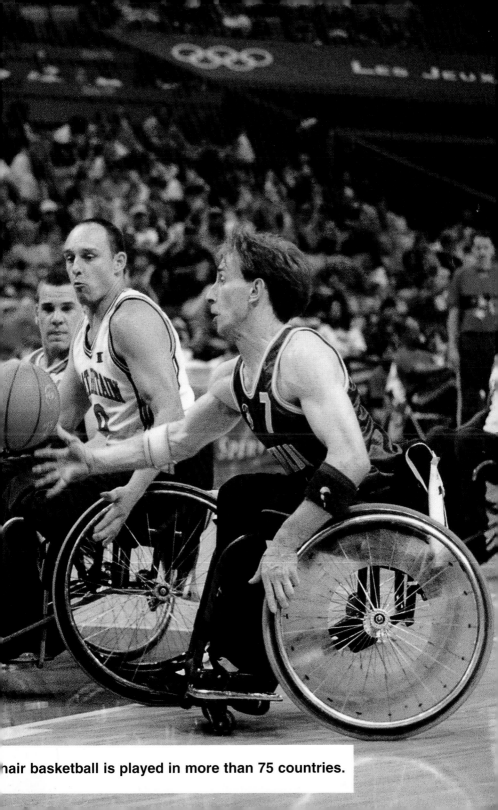

hair basketball is played in more than 75 countries.

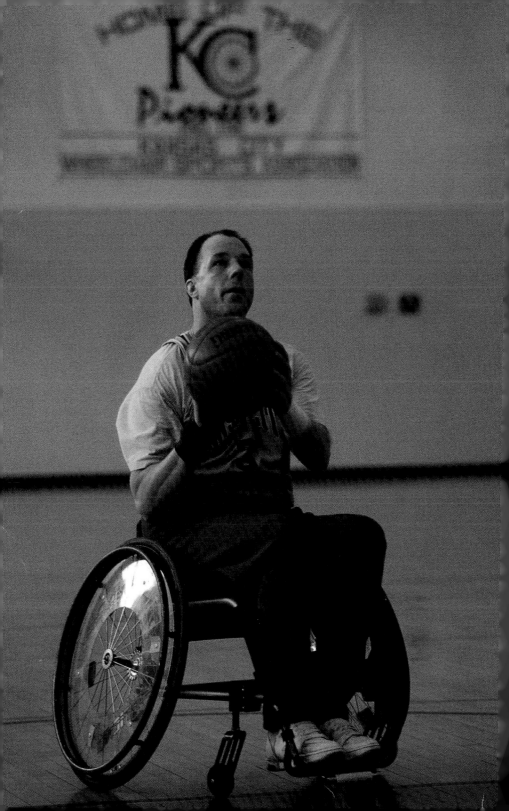

Chapter 2
History

After World War II, wheelchair patients returned to their communities. They taught other people with disabilities how to play wheelchair basketball. Some started hometown teams.

In 1949, six teams from the midwestern United States played in the first National Wheelchair Basketball Tournament. A tournament is a series of games played to find out which team is best. The team from Kansas City was called the Rolling Pioneers. The Rolling Pioneers won the first tournament. They beat the Minneapolis Rolling Gophers in the championship game.

The Kansas City Rolling Pioneers won the first wheelchair basketball tournament.

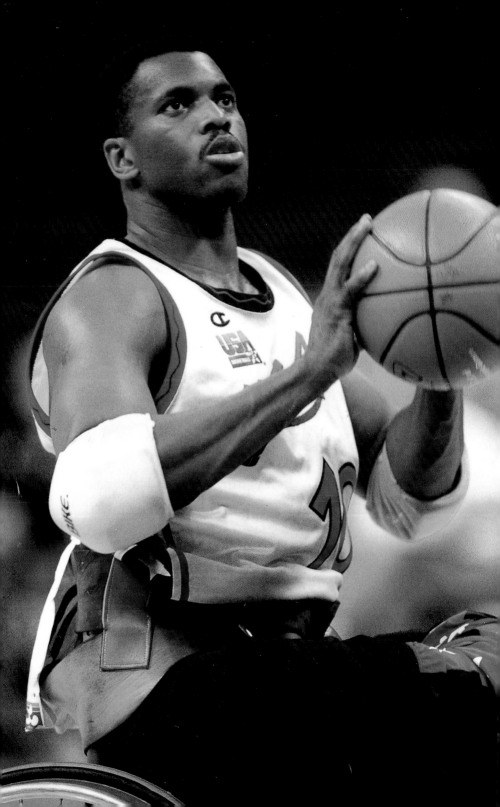

The NWBA

The same players decided to hold the National Wheelchair Basketball Tournament every year. They also formed the National Wheelchair Basketball Association (NWBA). The NWBA is in charge of wheelchair basketball in the United States.

Today, 187 teams are members of the NWBA. There are 139 men's teams, eight college teams, and 30 youth teams. There are youth teams for boys and for girls. The first Women's National Wheelchair Basketball Tournament was held in 1974. Ten women's teams are now members of the NWBA.

NWBA teams play in cities and towns throughout the United States. More than 2,500 people are registered to play.

NWBA Tournaments

For many years, the NWBA held just one tournament for men's teams each year. Teams tried to gather the best players from around the

More than 2,500 people are registered to play wheelchair basketball in the United States.

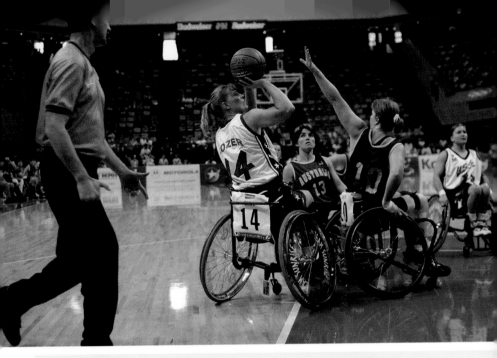

Both men's teams and women's teams compete in international tournaments.

country. A few teams paid the travel expenses of players from other towns. Because of the travel expenses, these players were rarely able to attend team practices. They practiced on their own.

In 1995, the NWBA created two divisions for the annual tournament. Division I teams can use wheelchair players from other areas. For example, a player who lives in Miami, Florida, can play for a team in Dallas, Texas. In this way, Division I teams are like professional basketball teams.

Division II teams far outnumber those in Division I. They are like hometown teams. All the players on a team come from the same town or area. These teams compete for the Division II national championship.

International Tournaments

Since 1976, the NWBA has formed national teams to compete in international tournaments. National teams are teams chosen to represent the country where the players live. International tournaments include teams from many countries.

The U.S. men's teams and women's teams have won many gold medals. Gold medals are awards given to the best team or the best athlete at a competition. U.S. teams have competed in the world championship, sometimes called the Gold Cup. The teams have also competed in the Paralympic Games.

Like the Olympic Games, the Paralympic Games are sports contests for athletes from many countries. However, all of the athletes at the Paralympic Games are people with disabilities. Both the Olympics and the Paralympics are held once every four years.

The Paralympics began in 1960. In the first 10 Paralympic Games, the U.S. men's team won five gold medals. The U.S. women's team first entered the Paralympics in 1968. The women's team won the gold medal in 1988.

Canadian Teams

Wheelchair basketball teams play in Canada, too. The Canadian Wheelchair Basketball Association (CWBA) started in 1986. The CWBA holds a national championship each year for men's and women's teams.

The women's national team from Canada has an outstanding record. The team won the gold medal at the 1992 and 1996 Paralympic Games. The team has been ranked the number one women's wheelchair team in the world.

The Canadian men's team won a silver medal in the 1986 world championship. Silver medals are awards given to the second-best team or the second-best athlete in a competition.

The U.S. women's team won a gold medal at the 1988 Paralymp

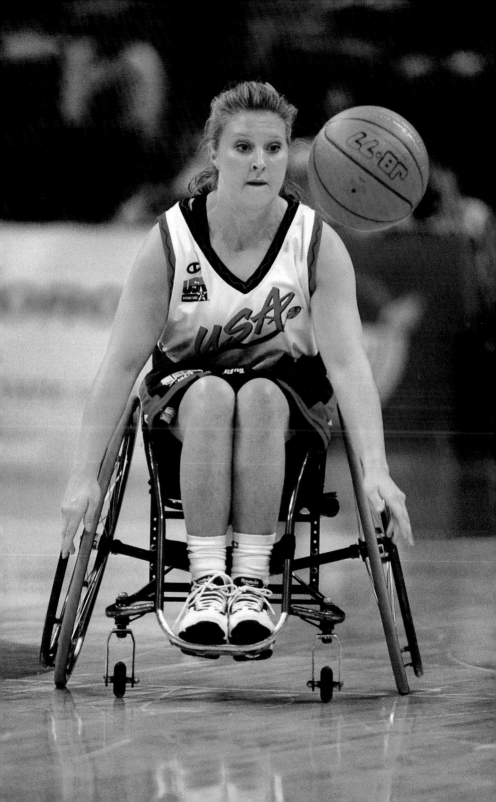

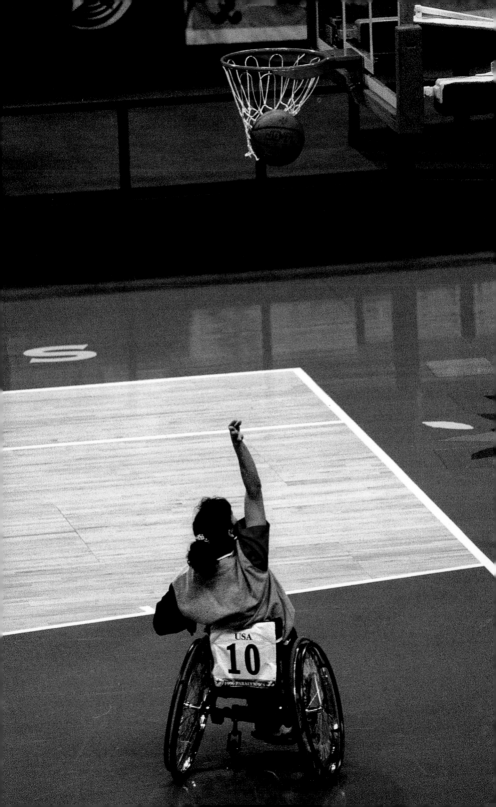

Chapter 3
The Players

Wheelchair basketball is played only by people with disabilities. Most are paraplegics. Paraplegics are people who have little or no ability to move the lower part of their bodies. Their disability can be caused by an injury, a disease, or a birth defect.

Practice

Wheelchair basketball players train and practice. They exercise to stay strong and healthy. They work to move their wheelchairs better and quicker. They practice passing, dribbling, and

Wheelchair players practice to improve their skills.

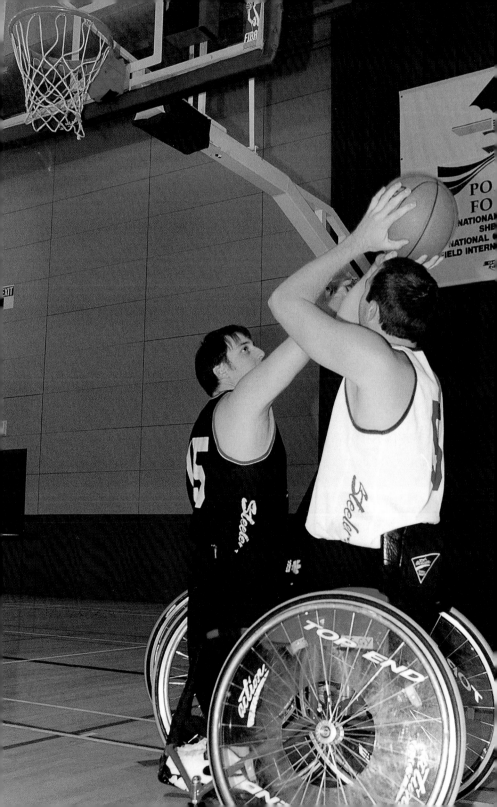

shooting baskets. Dribbling means using one hand to bounce a basketball off the floor.

Here is what often happens at a team practice. First, the players take several laps around the basketball court in their wheelchairs. Then they work on their passing and shooting skills. They practice driving toward the basket and shooting from close-up. They shoot the ball off the backboard and into the basket. This shot is called a layup.

The coach puts the players through drills. Drills are exercises repeated over and over to practice a skill. During some drills, teams practice dribbling, passing, and shooting baskets. During other drills, they practice keeping other players from scoring. Keeping the other team from scoring is called defense.

A practice may last two or three hours. It may end with a practice game, called a scrimmage.

Close-up shots that bounce off the backboard are called layups.

Who Can Play?

A player must have a permanent disability in one leg or both legs. A permanent disability is a disability that cannot be changed or cured. People with temporary disabilities are not allowed to play on wheelchair basketball teams.

Each wheelchair player is placed in one of three classes. A doctor or physical therapist decides which class is right for each player. A physical therapist is a person trained to help people with physical disabilities.

The Three Classes

Class I players are the most severely disabled. Their back and stomach muscles are paralyzed. Paralyzed means unable to move or feel. The athletes cannot move or feel their paralyzed muscles. They have poor sitting balance and cannot sit on their own without support. If they lean forward, they must use their arms to keep from falling. They can usually push themselves back into a wheelchair with their arms.

A doctor or physical therapist decides which class is right for each wheelchair player.

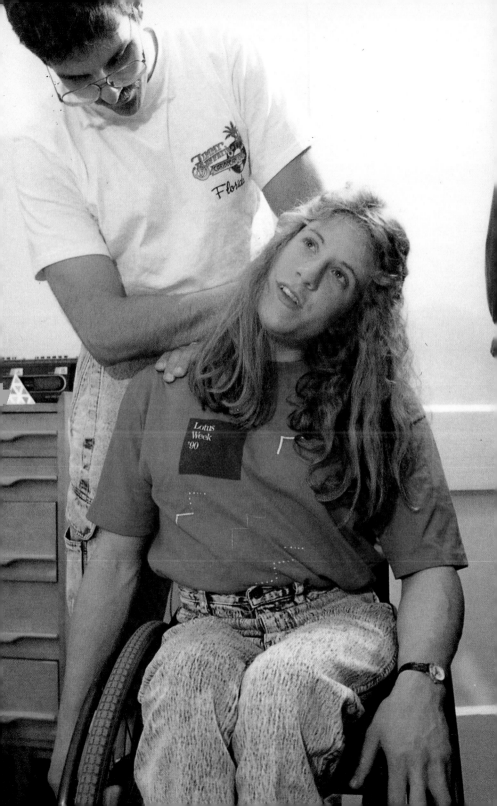

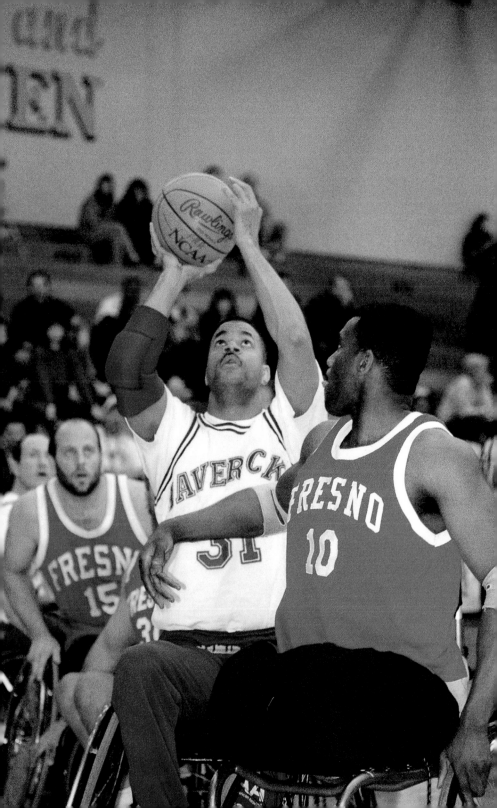

Class II players have some feeling in their back and stomach muscles. They have better sitting balance than Class I players. But they have little or no use of their legs and feet.

Class III players are the least disabled. Their stomach and back muscles are not paralyzed. They can sit without support. Most have some control over their leg and foot muscles. But some Class III players have had one or both legs removed. The removal of a leg or an arm is called amputation.

In 1964, the NWBA began using a team point system. The system is designed to give all athletes with disabilities a chance to play.

The system assigns points based on each player's class. A Class I player counts for one point. A Class II player counts for two points. Class III players count for three points.

During a game, each team puts five players on the court. The five players must add up to 12 points or less. No team can play more than two Class III players at one time.

The NWBA uses a point system so all athletes have a chance to play.

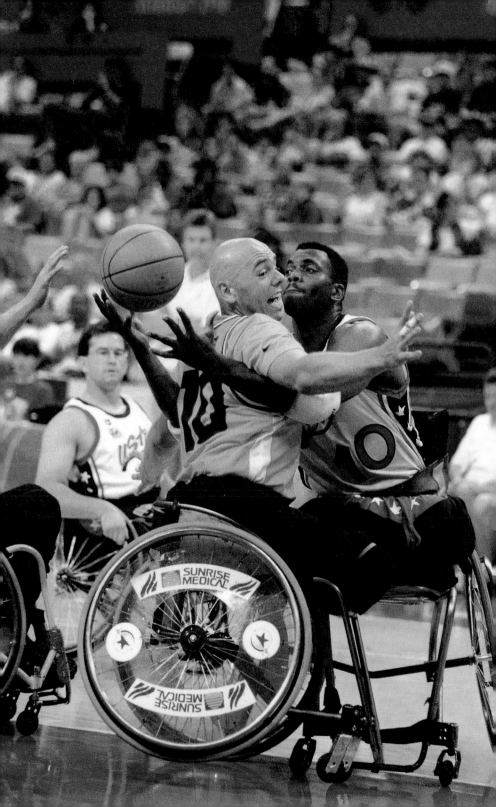

Chapter 4
Equipment and Safety

In the 1940s, manufacturers made wheelchairs out of steel and chrome. The chairs weighed 40 to 50 pounds (18 to 22 kilograms). They were hard to move because they were so heavy. They were not designed to let people with disabilities move around easily without help.

Wheelchair users had trouble playing sports in these heavy chairs. But after World War II, wheelchair athletes started to improve their own chairs. They made the wheelchair backs shorter and the armrests smaller. Now they could move their upper bodies more easily.

Wheelchairs must protect players during crashes.

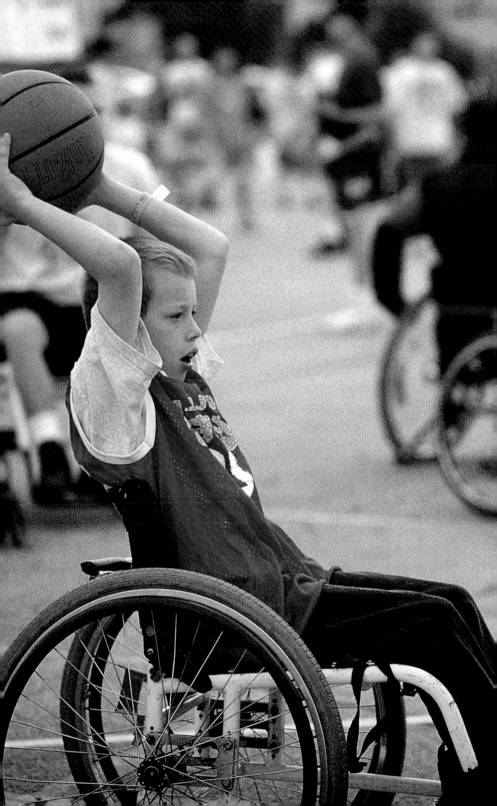

Later improvements made the chairs lighter and faster. Wheelchair basketball players learned how to race forward and turn quickly. They learned how to push their wheelchairs while dribbling the ball.

The Basketball Wheelchair

Today, some wheelchairs are made especially for basketball. The basketball chairs are made of materials that are lightweight but strong. The materials are similar to those used to make lightweight bicycles. Many chairs weigh less than 25 pounds (11 kilograms).

Because they are made of special materials, basketball wheelchairs are expensive. The average chair costs about $2,000.

A basketball wheelchair has bicycle-sized rear wheels. The wheelchair has one or two small front wheels called casters. Players rest their feet on foot rests at the front of the chairs. They use leg straps to hold their legs in place.

A basketball wheelchair has bicycle-sized rear wheels.

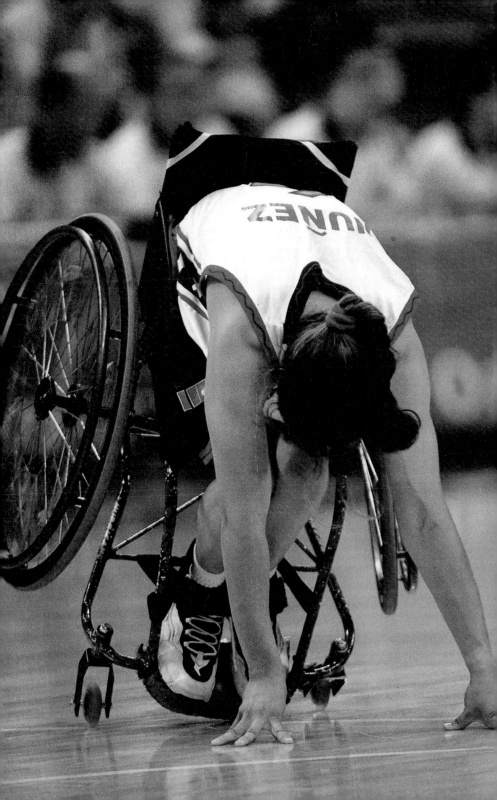

Players move their chairs by pushing on the handrims. A handrim is a metal tube or rim attached to the outside of each rear wheel. Each handrim is about one-half inch (one and one-quarter centimeters) wide.

Some basketball wheelchairs have armrests, but many players now prefer chairs without armrests. These chairs allow easy movement of the arms and upper body. Removing the armrests also makes the chairs lighter.

Safety

Today's wheelchairs are safer than the older chairs. Because they are made of strong metals, they rarely break. If a player tips over, the chair protects the player. Most players can put the chair back on its wheels without help.

Many players use straps to keep themselves in the wheelchair. The straps act like seat belts in cars. When the straps are used, a player who tips over stays in the wheelchair. Straps also help the player turn and move the chair more easily.

When straps are used, a player who tips over stays in the chair.

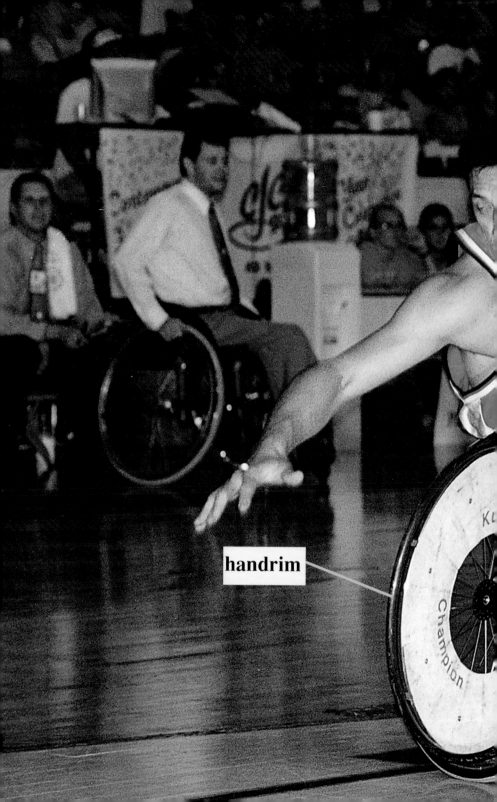

handrim

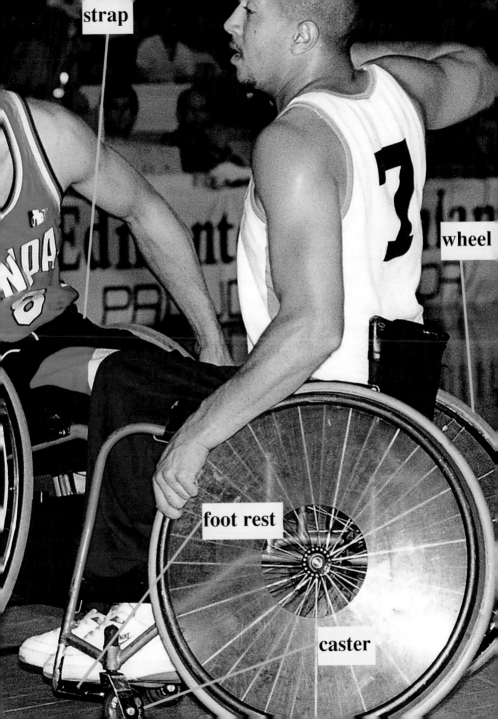

strap

wheel

foot rest

caster

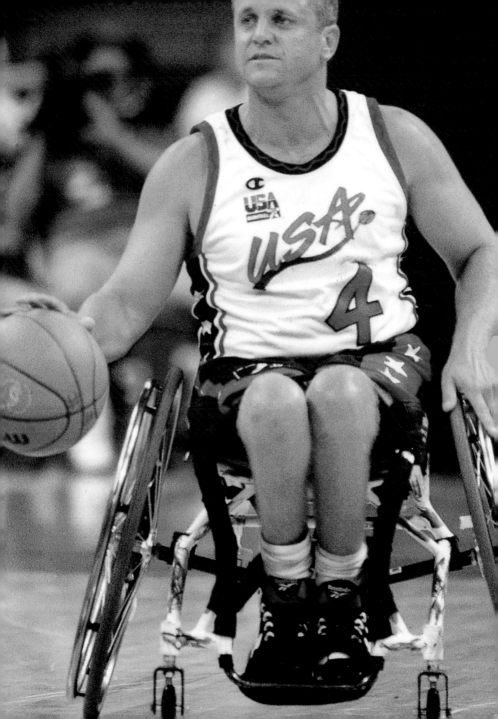

Chapter 5
The Rules

People with disabilities participate in many sports. Sometimes this requires changing the rules of the sport.

Wheelchair basketball was the first team sport for people with disabilities. It is played on a basketball court with a standard basketball. The height of the basket is not changed. Only a few rules are changed.

Dribbling

A wheelchair player can dribble in two ways. The player can place the ball on his or her lap. The player can then push the wheels of the chair once or twice to move it. After two pushes, the player must bounce the ball off the floor. Pushing the

A wheelchair player can dribble the ball in two ways.

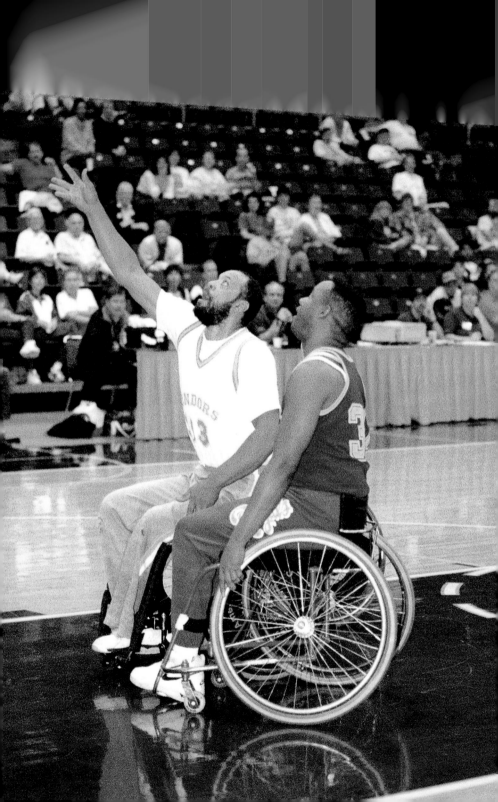

wheels three times in a row without dribbling is called a traveling violation. A violation is an action that breaks the rules of the game.

A player can also dribble with one hand while pushing the chair with the other. This is like a basketball dribble. It lets the player move and bounce the ball at the same time.

Lane Violations

The lane is a dark, rectangle-shaped area in front of the basket. In basketball, an offensive player can stay in the lane for only three seconds. An offensive player is any member of the team that has the ball.

In wheelchair basketball, an offensive player can stay in the lane for four seconds. The extra second gives players time to move around other wheelchairs. If a player stays in the lane for more than four seconds, it is a lane violation. The ball is given to the other team.

An offensive player can stay in the lane for four seconds.

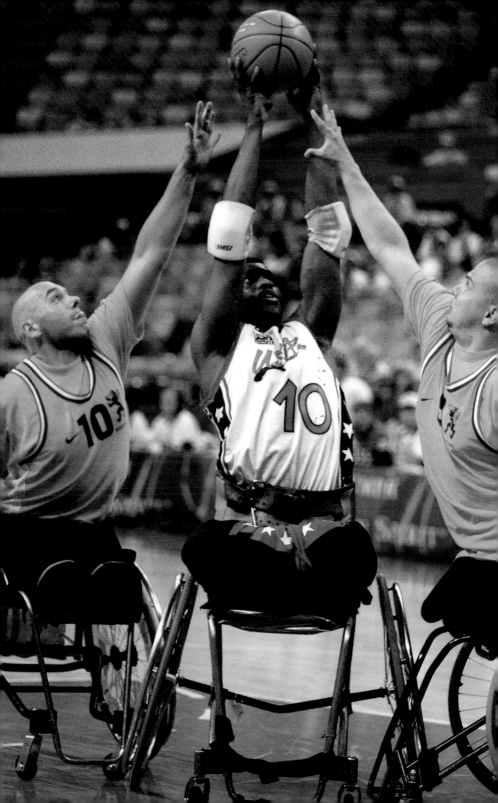

Other Violations

A player's wheelchair is not allowed to touch the boundary lines around the outside of the basketball court. If a player's chair touches the line, it is an out-of-bounds violation.

A player must stay seated in the wheelchair at all times. If a player rises from the chair, it is a physical advantage violation. The opposing team is awarded two free throws. This rule keeps players who have some use of their legs from gaining an advantage over others.

Teamwork

Wheelchair basketball is like basketball. Players need the same passing, shooting, and dribbling skills. The action is fast and exciting. Like any team sport, wheelchair basketball is built on teamwork, skill, and fun. Each athlete must also know and obey the rules of the game.

Wheelchair basketball is built on teamwork, skill, and fun.

Words to Know

amputation (am-pyuh-TAY-shun)—the removal of an arm or a leg

backboard (BAK-bord)—a board placed behind the basketball hoop

dribble (DRIB-uhl)—to bounce a basketball off the floor using one hand

drill (DRIL)—an exercise repeated over and over to practice a skill

handrims (HAND-rims)—metal tubes or rims attached to the outside of a wheelchair's rear wheels

lane (LAYN)—the dark, rectangle-shaped area in front of the basket

layup (LAY-uhp)—a basketball shot; the player with the ball moves toward the basket and shoots from close-up, bouncing the ball off the backboard

national team (NASH-uh-nuhl TEEM)—a team chosen to represent the country where the players live

offensive player (uh-FEN-siv PLAY-ur)—a member of the team that has the ball

Olympic Games (oh-LIM-pik GAMES)—sports contests for teams from many countries; held every four years

Paralympic Games (pa-ruh-LIM-pik GAMES)—games like the Olympic Games for athletes with disabilities; held every four years

paraplegic (pa-ruh-PLEE-jik)—a person who has little or no ability to move the lower half of the body

paralyzed (PA-ruh-lized)—unable to move or feel

physical therapist (FIZ-uh-kuhl THER-uh-pist)—a person trained to help people with physical disabilities

scrimmage (SKRIM-ij)—a practice game

tournament (TUR-nuh-muhnt)—a series of games played to find out which team is best

violation (vye-oh-LAY-shun)—an action that breaks the rules of a sport or game

To Learn More

Hedrick, Brad, Dan Byrnes, and Lew Shaver. *Wheelchair Basketball*. Washington, D.C.: Paralyzed Veterans of America, 1994.

Matthewman, Jim. *Basketball*. New York: Cambridge University Press, 1985.

Savitz, Harriet May. *Wheelchair Champions*. New York: Crowell, 1978.

Strohkendl, Horst. *The 50th Anniversary of Wheelchair Basketball*. New York: Waxmann Publishing, 1996.

Weisman, Marilee, and Jan Godfrey. *So Get on with It: A Celebration of Wheelchair Sports*. Toronto: Doubleday Canada, 1976.

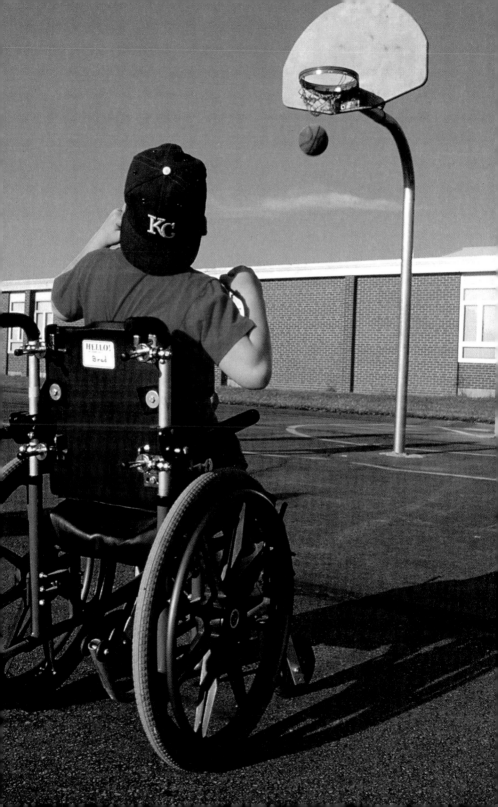

Useful Addresses

Canadian Wheelchair Basketball Association (CWBA)
1600 James Naismith Drive
Gloucester, ON
Canada K1B 5N4

International Wheelchair Basketball Federation (IWBF)
1 Meadow Close
Shavington, Crewe
Cheshire CW2 5BE
England

National Wheelchair Basketball Association (NWBA)
Office of the Commissioner
Charlotte Institute for Rehabilitation
1100 Blythe Blvd
Charlotte, NC 28203

***Sports 'N Spokes* magazine**
2111 East Highland Avenue
Suite 180
Phoenix, AZ 85106-4702

Wheelchair Sports USA (WSUSA)
3595 E. Fountain Boulevard
Suite L-1
Colorado Springs, CO 80910

Internet Sites

National Wheelchair Basketball Association
http://www.nwba.org:80compnotes.html

**USA Women's Wheelchair Basketball
  Homepage**
http://cwis.unomaha.edu/%7Ebrasile/usawomen.
  htm

Wheelchair Basketball
http://www.bbhighway.com/Events/1wheelchair.
  html

The World of Wheelchair Basketball
http://www.cwba.ca

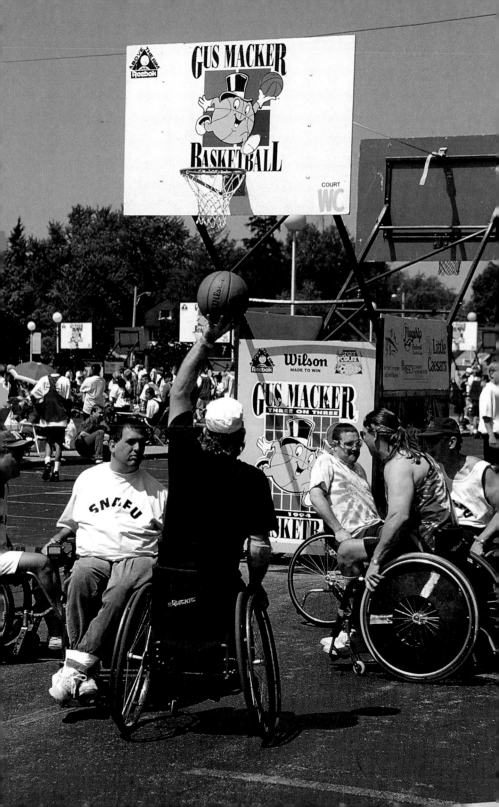

Index